Diabetic Gastroparesis Diet Cookbook

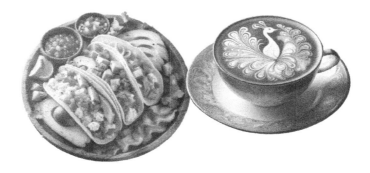

Improve Your Blood Sugar and Digestion with a Diabetic Gastroparesis-Friendly Diet

Lanita Cruz

Copyright © 2024 by Lanita Cruz

All rights reserved. No part of this publication may be reproduced, distributed, or transmitted in any form or by any means, including photocopying, recording, or other electronic or mechanical methods, without the prior written permission of the publisher, except in the case of brief quotations embodied in critical reviews and certain other noncommercial uses permitted by copyright law.

TABLE OF CONTENT

Introduction 7
CHAPTER 1 9
   Principles of the Diabetic Gastroparesis Diet 9
   Benefits of Diabetic Gastroparesis Diet 10
   Foods to Eat 12
   Foods to Avoid 14
   Comprehensive Shopping List for Diabetic Gastroparesis Diet 16
   Breakfast Recipes for Diabetic Gastroparesis Diet 18
   White Cheddar Zucchini Muffins 18
   Meyer Lemon Avocado Toast 20
   Crustless Quiche 22
   Mushroom Freezer Breakfast Burritos 24
   Scallion Grits With Shrimp 26
   Mini Corn, Cheese, and Basil Frittatas 28
   Vegetarian Eggs and Lentils on Toast 30
   Lunch Recipes for Diabetic Gastroparesis Diet 32
   Tuna Teriyaki Kabobs 32
   Garlic Tilapia with Spicy Kale 34
   Shrimp Orzo with Feta 35
   Fish Tacos with Guacamole 37
   Caprese Sandwich 40
   Artichoke Ratatouille Chicken 42
   Egg Salad Lettuce Wraps 44
   Dinner Recipes for Diabetic Gastroparesis Diet 46

Feta Garbanzo Bean Salad 46
Skillet Sea Scallops 48
Carne Asada Tacos 49
Green Goddess Salad with Chickpeas 52
Asian Lettuce Wraps 54
Beef and Spinach Lo Mein 56
Hamburger Vegetable Soup 58
Desserts and Snacks for Diabetic Gastroparesis Diet 60
Root Beer Float Pie 60
Tropical Mango Popsicles 62
Peppermint Meringues 64
Low-Carb Trail Mix 65
Ginger Plum Tart 67
Beverages/Drinks for Diabetic Gastroparesis Diet 68
Cinny Tea 68
Pumpkin Latte 70
Mojito Mocktails 71
Dandy Chai 73
Rooibos Tea 74

CHAPTER 3 77
30 Days Meal Plan For Diabetic Gastroparesis Diet 77

CHAPTER 4 87
Conclusion 87

Disclaimer

The information provided in this cookbook is for educational and informational purposes only. It is not intended to be a substitute for professional medical advice, diagnosis, or treatment.

Always seek the advice of your physician or other qualified health provider with any questions you may have regarding a medical condition.

The recipes and dietary suggestions included are based on general principles and may not be suitable for everyone.

Individual dietary needs and health conditions vary, and it is essential to consult with a healthcare professional before making significant changes to your diet.

The author and publisher disclaim responsibility for any effects resulting directly or indirectly from the use or misuse of the information provided in this cookbook.

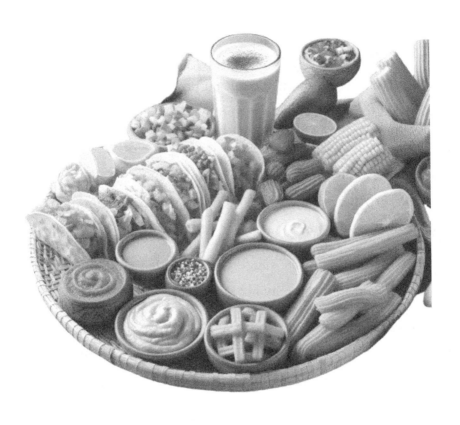

Introduction

Welcome to the "Diabetic Gastroparesis Diet Cookbook," your essential guide to managing diabetic gastroparesis through a carefully curated collection of delicious and gastroparesis-friendly recipes.

This cookbook is designed to empower individuals navigating the challenges of diabetes and gastroparesis, offering not just a collection of recipes but also insights into the principles of the Diabetic Gastroparesis Diet.

As you embark on this culinary journey, discover the benefits of embracing a diet tailored to address the unique needs of those with gastroparesis.

From detailed food lists to a comprehensive shopping guide, this cookbook equips you with the knowledge to make informed choices.

Whether you're planning breakfast, lunch, dinner, or satisfying your sweet tooth with desserts and snacks, each recipe is crafted to nourish and delight. Additionally, find a variety of beverages that align with the Diabetic Gastroparesis Diet.

To kickstart your journey, we've included a 30-day meal plan sample, providing a roadmap for balanced and flavorful eating.

Join us in exploring the intersection of health and culinary pleasure as we embark on this transformative culinary adventure.

CHAPTER 1
Principles of the Diabetic Gastroparesis Diet

1. **Low-Fiber, Easily Digestible Foods:** The diet prioritizes low-fiber options to ease digestion, minimizing the risk of exacerbating gastroparesis symptoms. Easily digestible foods ensure a gentler transit through the digestive system.
2. **Small, Frequent Meals**: Rather than large, infrequent meals, the focus is on consuming smaller portions at more frequent intervals. This helps regulate blood sugar levels and reduces the strain on the digestive system.
3. **Balanced Nutrient Intake:** A well-rounded mix of macronutrients, including carbohydrates, proteins, and healthy fats, is emphasized. This balance contributes to sustained energy levels and supports overall health.
4. **Mindful Carbohydrate Choices**: The diet encourages choosing carbohydrates wisely, favoring complex carbohydrates over simple sugars. This

approach helps in managing blood sugar levels and mitigating potential spikes.
5. **Hydration:** Staying adequately hydrated is vital. The principles recommend mindful consumption of fluids between meals to prevent excessive fullness during eating, a common challenge for individuals with gastroparesis.
6. **Individualized Approach**: Recognizing that each person's experience with gastroparesis is unique, the principles emphasize the importance of tailoring the diet to individual needs and tolerances. This encourages readers to experiment and find what works best for them.

Benefits of Diabetic Gastroparesis Diet

1. **Symptom Management**: By adhering to the Diabetic Gastroparesis Diet, you can experience improved symptom management. This includes reduced nausea, bloating, and discomfort associated with gastroparesis, contributing to an enhanced quality of life.
2. **Stabilized Blood Sugar Levels**: One of the primary advantages of this diet is its impact on blood sugar

control. Through mindful food choices, you can better regulate your blood glucose levels, minimizing fluctuations and promoting overall metabolic health.

3. **Enhanced Digestive Comfort**: The emphasis on easily digestible, low-fiber foods supports a more comfortable digestive process. This can alleviate the burden on the digestive system and mitigate symptoms such as delayed stomach emptying.

4. **Energy Balance**: The balanced distribution of macronutrients in the Diabetic Gastroparesis Diet helps maintain steady energy levels throughout the day. This ensures that you receive the necessary nutrients without overwhelming their digestive system.

5. **Improved Nutrient Absorption**: The focus on nutrient-dense foods enhances the absorption of essential vitamins and minerals. This is particularly important, as compromised digestion can impact the body's ability to extract nutrients from food.

6. **Weight Management**: The diet provides a structured approach to caloric intake, helping you achieve and maintain a healthy weight.
7. **Empowerment Through Knowledge**: This section empowers you by imparting a deeper understanding of how dietary choices impact your health. Armed with this knowledge, you can make informed decisions that align with their unique needs and preferences.

Foods to Eat

- **Lean Proteins**: Incorporate lean protein sources like poultry, tofu, fish, and legumes. These options provide essential amino acids for muscle health without overburdening the digestive system.
- **Soft Cooked Vegetables**: Opt for well-cooked, low-fiber vegetables like carrots, zucchini, and spinach. These choices ensure a nutrient-rich addition to meals while being gentle on the digestive tract.
- **Ripe Fruits**: Choose ripe fruits that are lower in fiber, such as bananas, melons, and peeled apples.

These fruits contribute natural sweetness and essential vitamins without causing undue stress on digestion.

- **White Grains and Starches:** Embrace white rice, pasta, and bread as staples. These easily digestible carbohydrates provide a steady source of energy while minimizing the risk of gastrointestinal discomfort.
- **Low-Fat Dairy**: Include low-fat dairy products like yogurt and milk in moderation. These items offer calcium and protein without the excess fat that may be harder to digest.
- **Nut Butters**: Nut butters, such as almond or peanut butter, are excellent sources of healthy fats and proteins. Spread them on soft crackers or incorporate them into smoothies for a satisfying snack.
- **Soups and Broths**: Warm soups and broths made with easily digestible ingredients are not only comforting but also contribute to hydration and nutrition. Choose broth-based soups with well-cooked vegetables and lean proteins.

- **Eggs**: Eggs are a versatile and protein-rich option, whether scrambled, boiled, or incorporated into dishes, they provide essential nutrients and are generally well-tolerated.
- **Cooked Cereals**: Opt for cooked cereals like oatmeal, cream of wheat, or rice porridge. These soft and easily digestible grains serve as wholesome breakfast options.
- **Herbs and Spices**: Flavor meals with herbs and spices to enhance taste without adding excessive salt or sugar. Common choices include ginger, mint, and mild spices that contribute to an enjoyable dining experience.

Foods to Avoid

- **High-Fiber Foods:** Limit the consumption of high-fiber foods, including whole grains, bran, and raw vegetables. These can contribute to gastric distress and discomfort due to their slower digestion rates.
- **Tough or Stringy Meats:** Opt for lean and tender cuts of meat, avoiding tougher or stringy options.

Gravitate towards minced or ground meats, as they are generally easier to digest.

- **Raw Fruits with Skin:** Steer clear of fruits with tough skins, seeds, or high fiber content. Examples include berries, citrus fruits with membranes, and fruits with seeds, as these can exacerbate gastroparesis symptoms.
- **Cruciferous Vegetables:** Minimize the intake of cruciferous vegetables like broccoli, cauliflower, and Brussels sprouts. While nutrient-dense, these can be challenging to digest and may cause bloating and discomfort.
- **High-Fat Dairy:** Reduce the consumption of high-fat dairy products, such as full-fat milk, cream, and rich cheeses. These items can slow down digestion and lead to feelings of fullness.
- **Fried and Greasy Foods:** Avoid fried and greasy foods, which can be difficult for the stomach to process. Opt for cooking methods like baking, steaming, or grilling for a gentler impact on digestion.

- **Carbonated Drinks**: Minimize or eliminate carbonated beverages, as they can contribute to bloating and gas. Instead, choose still water or herbal teas to stay adequately hydrated.
- **High-Sugar Sweets:** Limit the intake of high-sugar sweets, candies, and desserts. Opt for sugar substitutes or recipes with controlled sugar content to manage blood sugar levels effectively.
- **Alcohol:** Reduce or eliminate alcohol consumption, as it can slow down digestion and may interact with medications. If consumed, do so in moderation and consult with healthcare professionals.
- **Spicy Foods:** Cut back on spicy foods, as they may trigger gastric discomfort and reflux. Opt for milder herbs and spices to flavor meals without causing irritation.

Comprehensive Shopping List for Diabetic Gastroparesis Diet

Proteins:

- Skinless poultry (chicken or turkey)

- Lean cuts of beef or pork (ground or minced)
- Fish (e.g., salmon, tilapia)
- Tofu or tempeh
- Eggs

Vegetables (Low-Fiber and Well-Cooked):

- Carrots
- Zucchini
- Spinach
- Bell peppers (seeded)
- Cucumbers (peeled)

Fruits (Ripe and Low-Fiber):

- Bananas
- Melons (cantaloupe, honeydew)
- Peeled apples
- Pears (peeled and soft)
- Avocados

Grains and Starches (White and Refined):

- White rice
- Pasta (white or refined)

- White bread or wraps
- Oatmeal
- Quinoa (in moderation)

Dairy (Low-Fat Options):

- Low-fat yogurt
- Skim or low-fat milk
- Cottage cheese (low-fat)
- Hard cheeses (in moderation)

Nut Butters:

- Almond butter
- Peanut butter

Herbs and Spices:

- Ginger
- Mint
- Cinnamon
- Basil
- Oregano

Breakfast Recipes for Diabetic Gastroparesis Diet

White Cheddar Zucchini Muffins

- **Preparation Time:** 20 minutes
- **Serves:** 12 muffins

Ingredients:

- 2 cups shredded zucchini
- 1 cup sharp white cheddar cheese, grated
- 1 1/2 cups all-purpose flour
- 1/2 cup whole wheat flour
- 1 teaspoon baking powder
- 1/2 teaspoon baking soda
- 1/2 teaspoon salt
- 1/4 teaspoon black pepper
- 2 large eggs
- 1/2 cup unsalted butter, melted
- 1/2 cup plain Greek yogurt
- 1 tablespoon Dijon mustard
- 1 tablespoon fresh chives, chopped

Nutritional Information: Calories: 180 | Protein: 7g | Carbohydrates: 15g | Fat: 10g | Fiber: 2g

Instructions:

1. Preheat the oven to 375°F (190°C) and grease a muffin tin.
2. Remove excess moisture from shredded zucchini by squeezing it with a kitchen towel.
3. In a large bowl, combine flours, baking powder, baking soda, salt, and black pepper.
4. In another bowl, whisk eggs, melted butter, Greek yogurt, and Dijon mustard.
5. Add the wet ingredients to the dry mixture, stirring until it is just combined.
6. Fold in shredded zucchini, white cheddar, and chopped chives.
7. Spoon the batter into muffin cups, filling each about two-thirds full.
8. Bake for 18-20 minutes or until a toothpick comes out clean.
9. Allow the muffins to cool for 5 minutes before transferring to a wire rack.

Serving Suggestions:

- Enjoy these savory muffins warm, paired with a light salad or as a side to your favorite soup. They make a delightful addition to brunch or a quick grab-and-go breakfast.

Meyer Lemon Avocado Toast

- **Preparation Time**: 10 minutes
- **Serves:** 2

Ingredients:

- 2 ripe avocados
- 4 slices whole-grain bread
- 1 Meyer lemon, zest, and juice
- 1 tablespoon extra-virgin olive oil
- Salt and black pepper to taste
- Red pepper flakes (optional, for garnish)
- Fresh cilantro or microgreens (optional, for garnish)

Nutritional Information: Calories: 280 | Protein: 6g | Carbohydrates: 24g | Fat: 19g | Fiber: 10g

Instructions:

1. Toast the slices of whole-grain bread to your preference.
2. While the bread is toasting, halve and pit the avocados, then scoop the flesh into a bowl.
3. Mash the avocado with a fork until you achieve your desired level of smoothness.
4. Add the zest and juice of the Meyer lemon to the mashed avocado, mixing well.
5. Drizzle extra-virgin olive oil into the avocado mixture and season with salt and black pepper to taste. Mix again.
6. Once the bread is toasted, spread the lemony avocado mixture evenly over each slice.
7. Optional: Garnish with red pepper flakes for a hint of heat and fresh cilantro or microgreens for added freshness.
8. Serve immediately and enjoy this vibrant and nutritious Meyer Lemon Avocado Toast.

Serving Suggestions:

- Pair this delightful avocado toast with a side of poached eggs for a protein boost, or serve it alongside a simple green salad for a light and satisfying breakfast.

Crustless Quiche

- **Preparation Time:** 30 minutes
- **Serves:** 6

Ingredients:

- 1 cup fresh spinach, chopped
- 1/2 cup cherry tomatoes, halved
- 1/2 cup bell peppers, diced
- 1/2 cup mushrooms, sliced
- 1 cup feta cheese, crumbled
- 6 large eggs
- 1 cup milk (skim or low-fat)
- 1 teaspoon olive oil
- 1/2 teaspoon dried oregano
- Salt and black pepper to taste
- Cooking spray for greasing

Nutritional Information: Calories: 190 | Protein: 14g | Carbohydrates: 6g | Fat: 12g | Fiber: 1g

Instructions:

1. Preheat the oven to 375°F (190°C) and grease a pie dish with cooking spray.
2. In a skillet, heat olive oil over medium heat, sauté spinach, cherry tomatoes, bell peppers, and mushrooms until softened. Set aside to cool.
3. In a large bowl, whisk together eggs, milk, dried oregano, salt, and black pepper.
4. Add the crumbled feta cheese to the egg mixture and stir to combine.
5. Spread the sautéed vegetables evenly in the greased pie dish.
6. Pour the egg and feta mixture over the vegetables.
7. Bake in the preheated oven for 25-30 minutes or until the quiche is set and golden brown.
8. Allow the quiche to cool for a few minutes before slicing.

Serving Suggestions:

- Serve this crustless quiche warm for breakfast or brunch. Pair it with a side salad or whole-grain toast for a complete and satisfying meal. This versatile dish is also excellent for make-ahead breakfasts or quick, protein-packed lunches.

Mushroom Freezer Breakfast Burritos

- **Preparation Time:** 30 minutes
- **Serves:** 8 burritos

Ingredients:

- 8 large eggs
- 1 cup mushrooms, sliced
- 1/2 cup red bell pepper, diced
- 1/2 cup green onions, chopped
- 1 cup of black beans (rinsed and drained)
- 1 cup shredded cheddar cheese
- 8 whole-grain or low-carb tortillas
- 1 tablespoon olive oil
- 1 teaspoon cumin
- Salt and black pepper to taste
- Salsa and Greek yogurt (for serving)

Nutritional Information: Calories: 280 | Protein: 15g | Carbohydrates: 25g | Fat: 13g | Fiber: 6g

Instructions:

1. In a skillet, heat olive oil over medium heat, add your mushrooms, bell pepper, and green onions. Sauté until vegetables are tender. Set aside.
2. In a bowl, whisk eggs and season with cumin, salt, and black pepper.
3. Scramble the eggs in the same skillet until just cooked through.
4. Warm your tortillas in the microwave or on a griddle.
5. Assemble the burritos by placing a spoonful of scrambled eggs on each tortilla.
6. Top with the sautéed vegetable mixture, black beans, and shredded cheddar cheese.
7. Fold the sides of the tortilla over the filling and then roll it up tightly.
8. Allow the burritos to cool, then wrap each one in parchment paper and foil for freezing.

Serving Suggestions:

- To enjoy, reheat the frozen burritos in the microwave for a quick and hearty breakfast. Serve with salsa and a dollop of Greek yogurt for added flavor. These freezer-friendly burritos make meal prep a breeze, providing a convenient and nutritious option for busy mornings.

Scallion Grits With Shrimp

- **Preparation Time:** 25 minutes
- **Serves**: 4

Ingredients:

- 1 cup stone-ground grits
- 4 cups water
- 1 cup sharp cheddar cheese, grated
- 1/2 cup scallions, finely chopped
- 1 pound large shrimp, peeled and deveined
- 2 tablespoons olive oil
- 3 cloves garlic, minced
- 1 teaspoon smoked paprika
- Salt and black pepper to taste
- Fresh parsley (for garnish)

Nutritional Information: Calories: 380 | Protein: 28g | Carbohydrates: 30g | Fat: 16g | Fiber: 2g

Instructions:

1. In a saucepan, bring water to a boil, slowly whisk in the grits and reduce heat to low. Cook, stirring occasionally, until thickened.
2. Stir in cheddar cheese and chopped scallions until it is well combined, then set aside.
3. Season shrimp with smoked paprika, salt, and black pepper.
4. In a skillet, heat olive oil over medium-high heat. Add minced garlic and sauté until fragrant.
5. Add seasoned shrimp to the skillet and cook until pink and opaque, about 2-3 minutes per side.
6. Serve the shrimp over a bed of scallion grits, garnished with fresh parsley.

Serving Suggestions:

- Pair this Scallion Grits with Shrimp dish with a side of steamed vegetables or a crisp green salad for a wholesome meal. The creamy grits complement the savory shrimp, creating a delightful combination of flavors and textures. This recipe is perfect for a comforting breakfast

Mini Corn, Cheese, and Basil Frittatas

- **Preparation Time:** 20 minutes
- **Serves:** 6

Ingredients:

- 6 large eggs
- 1/2 cup corn kernels (fresh or frozen)
- 1/2 cup cheddar cheese, shredded
- 1/4 cup fresh basil, finely chopped
- 1/4 cup milk (skim or low-fat)
- 1 tablespoon olive oil
- 1/2 teaspoon baking powder
- Salt and black pepper to taste
- Cooking spray for greasing

Nutritional Information: Calories: 140 | Protein: 9g | Carbohydrates: 4g | Fat: 10g | Fiber: 1g

Instructions:

1. Preheat the oven to 375°F (190°C) and grease a mini-muffin tin with cooking spray.

2. In a skillet, heat olive oil over medium heat, add corn kernels and sauté until slightly golden. Set aside.
3. In a bowl, whisk together eggs, milk, baking powder, salt, and black pepper until well combined.
4. Stir in shredded cheddar cheese, fresh basil, and sautéed corn into the egg mixture.
5. Pour the mixture evenly into the mini-muffin tin, filling each cup about two-thirds full.
6. Bake in the preheated oven for 12-15 minutes or until the frittatas are set and lightly golden.
7. Allow the mini frittatas to cool for a few minutes before removing them from the tin.

Serving Suggestions:

- Serve these Mini Corn, Cheese, and Basil Frittatas as a delightful breakfast or brunch option. They are also perfect for a light snack. Pair with a side of fresh fruit or a small green salad for a balanced and satisfying meal.

Vegetarian Eggs and Lentils on Toast

- **Preparation Time:** 15 minutes

- Serves: 2

Ingredients:

- 4 large eggs
- 1 cup cooked lentils (canned or pre-cooked)
- 2 slices whole-grain bread
- 1 cup cherry tomatoes, halved
- 1/2 cup feta cheese, crumbled
- 1 tablespoon olive oil
- 1 teaspoon cumin
- Salt and black pepper to taste
- Fresh parsley (for garnish)

Nutritional Information: Calories: 380 | Protein: 24g | Carbohydrates: 30g | Fat: 18g | Fiber: 9g

Instructions:

1. Toast the slices of whole-grain bread according to your preference.
2. In a skillet, heat olive oil over medium heat, add cooked lentils, cherry tomatoes, and cumin. Sauté until tomatoes are softened.

3. Create wells in the lentil mixture and crack eggs into each well.
4. Cook until the egg whites are set but the yolks are still runny, season with salt and black pepper to taste.
5. Place the lentil and egg mixture on top of the toasted bread slices.
6. Sprinkle crumbled feta cheese over each toast and garnish with fresh parsley.

Serving Suggestions:

- Serve these Vegetarian Eggs and Lentils on Toast for a protein-packed and satisfying breakfast. Pair with a side of mixed greens or avocado slices for an extra dose of nutrients. This recipe offers a flavorful and nutritious option for those looking for a plant-based twist on traditional eggs on toast.

Lunch Recipes for Diabetic Gastroparesis Diet

Tuna Teriyaki Kabobs

- **Preparation Time**: 25 minutes

- **Serves**: 4

Ingredients:

- 1 pound of fresh tuna, diced into cubes
- 1/2 cup low-sodium soy sauce
- 2 tablespoons honey
- 1 tablespoon olive oil
- 2 cloves garlic, minced
- 1 teaspoon ginger, grated
- 1 tablespoon sesame seeds (optional)
- Fresh cilantro or green onions (for garnish)
- Skewers, soaked in water

Nutritional Information: Calories: 220 | Protein: 25g | Carbohydrates: 9g | Fat: 9g | Fiber: 0.5g

Instructions:

1. In a bowl, whisk together soy sauce, honey, olive oil, minced garlic, and grated ginger to create the teriyaki marinade.
2. Place the tuna cubes in a shallow dish and pour half of the teriyaki marinade over them. Let it marinate for 15-20 minutes.

3. Preheat the grill or grill pan over medium-high heat, thread the marinated tuna cubes onto the skewers.
4. Grill the tuna kabobs for 2-3 minutes per side or until desired doneness, basting with the remaining teriyaki marinade.
5. Optional: Sprinkle sesame seeds and garnish with fresh cilantro or green onions before serving.

Serving Suggestions:

- Serve the Tuna Teriyaki Kabobs over a bed of steamed brown rice. Add a side of sautéed vegetables or a light salad for a well-balanced meal. These kabobs are perfect for a healthy and flavorful lunch option.

Garlic Tilapia with Spicy Kale

- **Preparation Time:** 30 minutes
- **Serves:** 2

Ingredients:

- 2 tilapia fillets
- 3 cups kale, chopped
- 4 cloves garlic, minced

- 1 tablespoon olive oil
- 1/2 teaspoon red pepper flakes
- Salt and black pepper to taste
- Lemon wedges (for garnish)

Nutritional Information: Calories: 250 | Protein: 28g | Carbohydrates: 8g | Fat: 12g | Fiber: 3g

Instructions:

1. Season the tilapia fillets with salt, black pepper, and half of the minced garlic.
2. In a skillet, heat olive oil over medium-high heat. Add the tilapia fillets and cook for 3-4 minutes per side or until cooked through, remove from the skillet and set aside.
3. In the same skillet, add the remaining minced garlic and red pepper flakes. Sauté for 1-2 minutes until fragrant.
4. Add chopped kale to the skillet, tossing to coat in the garlic-infused oil. Cook until the kale is wilted and slightly crispy on the edges.
5. Place the cooked tilapia fillets on a bed of spicy kale.

6. Optional: Garnish with additional red pepper flakes and serve with lemon wedges on the side.

Serving Suggestions:

- Pair Garlic Tilapia with Spicy Kale with a side of quinoa or cauliflower rice for a low-carb option. This dish is a delicious and nutritious choice for a quick and satisfying lunch or dinner. The combination of garlicky tilapia and spicy kale offers a burst of flavors and textures.

Shrimp Orzo with Feta

- **Preparation Time:** 25 minutes
- **Serves:** 4

Ingredients:

- 1 cup orzo pasta
- 1 pound shrimp, peeled and deveined
- 1 cup cherry tomatoes, halved
- 1/2 cup crumbled feta cheese
- 1/4 cup fresh parsley, chopped
- 3 tablespoons olive oil
- 2 cloves garlic, minced

- 1 teaspoon dried oregano
- Salt and black pepper to taste
- Lemon wedges (for serving)

Nutritional Information: Calories: 350 | Protein: 25g | Carbohydrates: 32g | Fat: 15g | Fiber: 2g

Instructions:

1. Cook orzo pasta according to package instructions, drain and set aside.
2. In a large skillet, heat olive oil over medium-high heat, add minced garlic and sauté until fragrant.
3. Add shrimp to the skillet and cook for 2-3 minutes per side or until they turn pink and opaque.
1. Stir in halved cherry tomatoes and dried oregano. Cook for an additional 2 minutes.
2. Add cooked orzo to the skillet, tossing to combine with the shrimp and tomatoes.
3. Season the dish with salt and black pepper to taste.
4. Sprinkle crumbled feta cheese over the shrimp and orzo mixture.
5. Garnish with fresh parsley and serve with lemon wedges on the side.

Serving Suggestions:

- Shrimp Orzo with Feta is a versatile dish that can be served hot or cold. Pair it with a side of mixed greens or a light cucumber salad for a refreshing touch. This recipe makes for a delightful lunch, offering a perfect balance of protein, carbs, and Mediterranean-inspired flavors.

Fish Tacos with Guacamole

- **Preparation Time:** 30 minutes
- **Serves:** 4

Ingredients:

- 1 pound white fish fillets (tilapia, cod, or your choice)
- 8 small corn tortillas
- 1 cup shredded cabbage
- 1 cup cherry tomatoes, diced
- 1/2 cup red onion, finely chopped
- 1/4 cup fresh cilantro, chopped
- 1 lime, cut into wedges

For the Fish Marinade:

- 2 tablespoons olive oil
- 1 teaspoon chili powder
- 1 teaspoon cumin
- 1/2 teaspoon garlic powder
- Salt and black pepper to taste

For the Guacamole:

- 2 ripe avocados, mashed
- 1 small tomato, diced
- 1/4 cup red onion, finely chopped
- 1 clove garlic, minced
- 1 tablespoon lime juice
- Salt and black pepper to taste

Nutritional Information: Calories: 280 | Protein: 20g | Carbohydrates: 28g | Fat: 12g | Fiber: 7g

Instructions:

1. In a bowl, mix together the ingredients for the fish marinade: olive oil, chili powder, cumin, garlic powder, salt, and black pepper.
2. Coat the fish fillets with the marinade and let them sit for 10 minutes.

3. In a grill pan or skillet, cook the fish fillets for 3-4 minutes per side or until they easily flake with a fork.
4. Warm the corn tortillas in the pan for about 20 seconds on each side.
5. In a separate bowl, prepare the guacamole by combining mashed avocados, diced tomato, chopped red onion, minced garlic, lime juice, salt, and black pepper.
6. Assemble the tacos by placing a portion of grilled fish on each tortilla.
7. Top with shredded cabbage, cherry tomatoes, red onion, and a dollop of guacamole.
8. Garnish with fresh cilantro and serve with lime wedges on the side.

Serving Suggestions:

- Serve these Fish Tacos with Guacamole with a side of black beans or a light slaw for a well-rounded meal. This recipe brings together the freshness of guacamole and the savory goodness of grilled fish for a delightful and satisfying lunch option.

Caprese Sandwich

- **Preparation Time:** 15 minutes
- **Serves:** 2

Ingredients:

- 4 slices whole-grain bread
- 2 large tomatoes, sliced
- 1 cup fresh mozzarella, sliced
- 1/4 cup fresh basil leaves
- 2 tablespoons balsamic glaze
- 1 tablespoon extra-virgin olive oil
- Salt and black pepper to taste

Nutritional Information: Calories: 380 | Protein: 18g | Carbohydrates: 32g | Fat: 20g | Fiber: 6g

Instructions:

1. Lay out the slices of whole-grain bread.
2. On two slices, evenly distribute the tomato slices.
3. Layer fresh mozzarella slices over the tomatoes.
4. Place fresh basil leaves on top of the mozzarella.
5. Drizzle balsamic glaze and extra-virgin olive oil over the basil.

6. Sprinkle with salt and black pepper to taste.
7. Top each sandwich with the remaining slices of bread to form sandwiches.
8. Optional: Grill the sandwiches on a panini press or in a skillet until the bread is toasted and the cheese is melted.

Serving Suggestions:

- Serve the Caprese Sandwiches with a side of mixed greens or a light cucumber salad. This recipe offers a classic combination of flavors with a healthy twist, making it an ideal choice for a quick and delicious lunch.

Artichoke Ratatouille Chicken

- **Preparation Time:** 35 minutes
- **Serves:** 4

Ingredients:

- 4 boneless, skinless chicken breasts
- 1 can (14 oz) of artichoke hearts (drained and quartered)
- 1 eggplant, diced

- 1 zucchini, diced
- 1 yellow bell pepper, diced
- 1 red onion, sliced
- 3 cloves garlic, minced
- 1 can (14 oz) diced tomatoes
- 2 tablespoons tomato paste
- 1 teaspoon dried thyme
- 1 teaspoon dried oregano
- 1/2 teaspoon dried rosemary
- Salt and black pepper to taste
- Fresh parsley (for garnish)

Nutritional Information: Calories: 320 | Protein: 30g | Carbohydrates: 18g | Fat: 15g | Fiber: 7g

Instructions:

1. Preheat the oven to 375°F (190°C).
2. Season chicken breasts with salt, black pepper, thyme, oregano, and rosemary.
3. In an oven-safe skillet, sear the chicken on both sides until golden brown. Remove and set aside.
4. In the same skillet, sauté garlic, onion, eggplant, zucchini, and bell pepper until softened.

5. Add diced tomatoes, tomato paste, and quartered artichoke hearts to the skillet. Stir well.
6. Place the seared chicken breasts on top of the vegetable mixture.
7. Transfer the skillet to the preheated oven and bake for 20-25 minutes or until the chicken is cooked through.
8. Garnish with fresh parsley before serving.

Serving Suggestions:

- The combination of artichokes, vibrant vegetables, and aromatic herbs creates a flavorful and satisfying dish. This recipe is perfect for a nutritious lunch option.

Egg Salad Lettuce Wraps

- **Preparation Time:** 15 minutes
- **Serves**: 2

Ingredients:

- 4 large eggs, hard-boiled and chopped
- 1/4 cup celery, finely diced
- 2 tablespoons red onion, finely chopped

- 2 tablespoons mayonnaise (preferably light)
- 1 teaspoon Dijon mustard
- Salt and black pepper to taste
- 4 large lettuce leaves (such as iceberg or butterhead)

Nutritional Information: Calories: 230 | Protein: 12g | Carbohydrates: 4g | Fat: 18g | Fiber: 1g

Instructions:

1. In a bowl, combine chopped hard-boiled eggs, diced celery, and finely chopped red onion.
2. In a small bowl, whisk together mayonnaise and Dijon mustard.
3. Add the mayo-mustard mixture to the egg mixture and stir until well combined.
4. Season the egg salad with salt and black pepper to taste. Adjust seasoning if needed.
5. Spoon the egg salad onto the center of each lettuce leaf.
6. Optional: Drizzle with additional mustard or sprinkle with paprika for extra flavor.
7. Fold the sides of the lettuce leaves over the egg salad to create wraps.

Serving Suggestions:

- Serve Egg Salad Lettuce Wraps as a light and refreshing lunch. Pair with a side of cherry tomatoes or cucumber slices for added freshness. These wraps are a low-carb alternative to traditional sandwiches, making them an excellent choice for a quick and satisfying meal.

Dinner Recipes for Diabetic Gastroparesis Diet

Feta Garbanzo Bean Salad

- **Preparation Time:** 15 minutes
- **Serves:** 4

Ingredients:

- 2 cans (15 oz each) garbanzo beans, drained and rinsed
- 1 cup cherry tomatoes, halved
- 1 cucumber, diced
- 1/2 red onion, finely chopped
- 1/2 cup crumbled feta cheese

- 1/4 cup Kalamata olives, pitted and sliced
- 2 tablespoons extra-virgin olive oil
- 1 tablespoon red wine vinegar
- 1 teaspoon dried oregano
- Salt and black pepper to taste
- Fresh parsley (for garnish)

Nutritional Information: Calories: 280 | Protein: 11g | Carbohydrates: 31g | Fat: 14g | Fiber: 9g

Instructions:

1. In a large mixing bowl, combine garbanzo beans, cherry tomatoes, cucumber, red onion, crumbled feta, and sliced Kalamata olives.
2. In a small bowl, whisk together olive oil, red wine vinegar, dried oregano, salt, and black pepper to create the dressing.
3. Pour the dressing over the salad ingredients and toss it until it is well coated.
4. Adjust seasoning if needed and let the salad marinate for a few minutes to enhance flavors.
5. Garnish with fresh parsley before serving.

Serving Suggestions:

- Serve Feta Garbanzo Bean Salad as a refreshing side dish or a light main course. Pair it with grilled chicken or fish for a complete meal. This salad is perfect for a quick and nutritious dinner, offering a delightful combination of textures and Mediterranean flavors.

Skillet Sea Scallops

- **Preparation Time:** 15 minutes
- **Serves:** 2

Ingredients:

- 1 pound sea scallops, patted dry
- 2 tablespoons olive oil
- 2 cloves garlic, minced
- 1 tablespoon unsalted butter
- 1 tablespoon fresh lemon juice
- 1 tablespoon chopped fresh parsley
- Salt and black pepper to taste
- Lemon wedges (for serving)

Nutritional Information: Calories: 220 | Protein: 25g | Carbohydrates: 3g | Fat: 12g | Fiber: 0.5g

Instructions:

1. Heat olive oil in a large skillet over medium-high heat until hot but not smoking.
2. Season sea scallops with salt and black pepper on both sides.
3. Carefully add scallops to the hot skillet, making sure they are not overcrowded.
4. Sear scallops for 1.5-2 minutes per side or until golden brown and opaque in the center.
5. Add minced garlic to the skillet and sauté for 30 seconds until fragrant.
6. Add unsalted butter to the skillet and let it melt, coating the scallops.
7. Drizzle fresh lemon juice over the scallops and sprinkle with chopped fresh parsley.
8. Remove from heat and serve immediately with lemon wedges on the side.

Serving Suggestions:

- Serve Skillet Sea Scallops over a bed of cauliflower rice or quinoa for a low-carb option. Pair with a side of steamed vegetables or a light salad. This quick and elegant dish is perfect for a special dinner, offering a burst of freshness and flavor.

Carne Asada Tacos

- **Preparation Time:** 30 minutes (plus marinating time)
- **Serves:** 4

Ingredients:

- 1.5 pounds flank or skirt steak
- 1/4 cup fresh orange juice
- 1/4 cup fresh lime juice
- 3 cloves garlic, minced
- 1 teaspoon ground cumin
- 1 teaspoon chili powder
- 1 teaspoon dried oregano
- Salt and black pepper to taste
- 8 small corn tortillas
- 1 cup diced onions
- 1 cup chopped cilantro
- Lime wedges (for serving)

Nutritional Information: Calories: 320 | Protein: 28g | Carbohydrates: 20g | Fat: 14g | Fiber: 3g

Instructions:

1. In a bowl, combine fresh orange juice, fresh lime juice, minced garlic, ground cumin, chili powder, dried oregano, salt, and black pepper to create the marinade.
2. Place the steak in a resealable plastic bag and pour the marinade over it, seal the bag and refrigerate for at least 2 hours or overnight.
3. Preheat a grill or grill pan over medium-high heat, remove the steak from the marinade and grill for 4-5 minutes per side or until desired doneness.
4. Let the steak rest for a few minutes before slicing it thinly against the grain.
5. Heat the corn tortillas on the grill or in a skillet until warm and pliable.
6. Assemble the tacos by placing slices of carne asada on each tortilla.
7. Top with diced onions and chopped cilantro, serve with lime wedges on the side.

Serving Suggestions:

- Serve Carne Asada Tacos with a side of black beans or a simple Mexican slaw. These tacos are perfect for a festive dinner, allowing everyone to customize their toppings. The marinated and grilled steak provides a burst of flavor that pairs well with the freshness of the toppings.

Green Goddess Salad with Chickpeas

- **Preparation Time:** 15 minutes
- **Serves:** 4

Ingredients:

- 6 cups of mixed salad greens (spinach, watercress, and arugula,)
- 15 oz (1 can) of chickpeas (rinsed and drained)
- 1 avocado, sliced
- 1 cucumber, sliced
- 1/2 cup cherry tomatoes, halved
- 1/4 cup pumpkin seeds (pepitas)
- 1/4 cup crumbled feta cheese (optional)
- Fresh basil and mint leaves for decorating

For the Green Goddess Dressing:

- 1/2 cup plain Greek yogurt
- 1/4 cup fresh parsley, chopped
- 2 tablespoons fresh tarragon, chopped
- 1 tablespoon chives, chopped
- 1 clove garlic, minced
- 2 tablespoons lemon juice
- Salt and black pepper to taste

Nutritional Information: Calories: 280 | Protein: 12g | Carbohydrates: 25g | Fat: 16g | Fiber: 8g

Instructions:

1. In a large salad bowl, combine mixed greens, chickpeas, avocado slices, cucumber slices, cherry tomatoes, and pumpkin seeds.
2. In a blender or food processor, combine Greek yogurt, fresh parsley, fresh tarragon, chives, minced garlic, lemon juice, salt, and black pepper. Blend until smooth to create the Green Goddess dressing.
3. Drizzle the Green Goddess dressing over the salad and toss gently to coat.
4. Top the salad with crumbled feta cheese, if desired.

5. Garnish with fresh basil and mint leaves.

Serving Suggestions:

- Serve Green Goddess Salad with Chickpeas as a light and satisfying dinner. Pair it with grilled chicken or salmon for added protein. This vibrant and nutrient-packed salad is not only delicious but also a visually appealing addition to your dinner table.

Asian Lettuce Wraps

- **Preparation Time**: 20 minutes
- **Serves**: 4

Ingredients:

- 1 pound ground chicken or turkey
- 2 tablespoons soy sauce (low-sodium)
- 1 tablespoon hoisin sauce
- 1 tablespoon sesame oil
- 2 teaspoons fresh ginger, minced

- 2 cloves garlic, minced
- 1 cup water chestnuts, finely chopped
- 1 cup shiitake mushrooms, finely chopped
- 1/4 cup green onions, chopped
- 1/4 cup cilantro, chopped
- 1 tablespoon rice vinegar
- 1 teaspoon Sriracha sauce (optional)
- 1 head iceberg or butter lettuce, leaves separated

Nutritional Information: Calories: 220 | Protein: 18g | Carbohydrates: 12g | Fat: 11g | Fiber: 3g

Instructions:

1. In a large skillet over medium heat, cook ground chicken or turkey until browned.
2. In a small bowl, whisk together soy sauce, hoisin sauce, and sesame oil.
3. Add minced ginger and garlic to the skillet, sautéing for 1-2 minutes until fragrant.
4. Stir in water chestnuts, shiitake mushrooms, and the soy sauce mixture. Cook for an additional 3-4 minutes.

5. Add green onions, cilantro, rice vinegar, and Sriracha sauce (if using). Stir to combine and cook for another 2 minutes.
6. Remove the skillet from heat and allow the mixture to cool slightly.
7. Spoon the Asian mixture into individual lettuce leaves, creating wraps.
8. Serve the Asian Lettuce Wraps with additional soy sauce or Sriracha on the side.

Serving Suggestions:

- These Asian Lettuce Wraps make for a light and flavorful dinner. Pair them with a side of steamed brown rice or quinoa for a complete meal. The combination of savory, sweet, and spicy flavors makes this dish a crowd-pleaser.

Beef and Spinach Lo Mein

- **Preparation Time:** 25 minutes
- **Serves**: 4

Ingredients:

- 8 oz whole wheat or egg noodles

- 1 pound lean beef sirloin, thinly sliced
- 2 tablespoons soy sauce (low-sodium)
- 1 tablespoon oyster sauce
- 1 tablespoon hoisin sauce
- 1 tablespoon sesame oil
- 2 teaspoons vegetable oil
- 3 cloves garlic, minced
- 1 tablespoon fresh ginger, grated
- 1 red bell pepper, thinly sliced
- 2 cups spinach leaves
- 2 green onions, sliced
- Sesame seeds for garnish (optional)

Nutritional Information: Calories: 380 | Protein: 28g | Carbohydrates: 40g | Fat: 14g | Fiber: 6g

Instructions:

1. Cook noodles according to package instructions. Drain and set aside.
2. In a bowl, marinate thinly sliced beef in soy sauce, oyster sauce, and hoisin sauce for 15 minutes.
3. Heat vegetable oil and sesame oil in a wok or large skillet over medium-high heat.

4. Add minced garlic and grated ginger, sautéing for 1-2 minutes until aromatic.
5. Add marinated beef to the wok, stirring continuously until cooked through and browned.
6. Toss in sliced red bell pepper and cook for an additional 2 minutes.
7. Add cooked noodles and spinach to the wok, tossing until the spinach wilts and the noodles are well-coated.
8. Garnish with sliced green onions and sesame seeds (if using).

Serving Suggestions:

- Serve Beef and Spinach Lo Mein hot, garnished with additional green onions and a sprinkle of sesame seeds. This quick and flavorful dish is a balanced combination of protein, vegetables, and noodles, making it an ideal choice for a satisfying dinner.

Hamburger Vegetable Soup

- **Preparation Time**: 30 minutes
- **Serves**: 6

Ingredients:

- 1 pound lean ground beef
- 1 onion, diced
- 2 carrots, peeled and sliced
- 2 celery stalks, sliced
- 2 cloves garlic, minced
- 1 can (14 oz) diced tomatoes
- 1 can (8 oz) tomato sauce
- 6 cups beef broth (low-sodium)
- 1 cup green beans, chopped
- 1 cup corn kernels (fresh or frozen)
- 1 cup peas (fresh or frozen)
- 2 teaspoons Italian seasoning
- Salt and black pepper to taste
- 2 cups baby spinach
- Fresh parsley for garnish

Nutritional Information: Calories: 280 | Protein: 20g | Carbohydrates: 20g | Fat: 12g | Fiber: 5g

Instructions:

1. In a large pot, brown the lean ground beef over medium-high heat until fully cooked.
2. Add diced onions, sliced carrots, sliced celery, and minced garlic to the pot. Sauté until vegetables are tender.
3. Pour in diced tomatoes, tomato sauce, and beef broth. Stir to combine.
4. Add chopped green beans, corn kernels, peas, Italian seasoning, salt, and black pepper. Bring the soup to a simmer.
5. Simmer for 15-20 minutes to allow flavors to meld and vegetables to soften.
6. Stir in baby spinach and cook until wilted.
7. Adjust seasoning if needed and serve hot, garnished with fresh parsley.

Serving Suggestions:

- Serve Hamburger Vegetable Soup with a side of whole-grain bread or a light salad. This hearty and nutritious soup is a comforting dinner option that combines the richness of beef with a variety of colorful vegetables.

Desserts and Snacks for Diabetic Gastroparesis Diet

Root Beer Float Pie

- **Preparation Time:** 20 minutes
- **Serves:** 8

Ingredients:

- 1 1/2 cups graham cracker crumbs
- 1/2 cup unsalted butter, melted
- 1 quart sugar-free vanilla ice cream, softened
- 1 cup diet root beer
- 1 package (0.3 oz) sugar-free vanilla instant pudding mix
- Whipped cream for topping (optional)

Nutritional Information: Calories: 250 | Protein: 5g | Carbohydrates: 30g | Fat: 14g | Fiber: 1g

Instructions:

1. In a bowl, combine graham cracker crumbs and melted butter. Press the mixture into the bottom of a pie dish to form the crust.

2. In a separate bowl, whisk together softened vanilla ice cream, diet root beer, and sugar-free vanilla instant pudding mix until well combined.
3. Pour the ice cream mixture into the prepared crust, spreading it evenly.
4. Freeze the pie for at least 4 hours or until firm.
5. Before serving, let the pie sit at room temperature for a few minutes to make slicing easier.
6. Optionally, top each slice with a dollop of whipped cream before serving.

Serving Suggestions:

- Serve Root Beer Float Pie chilled on a warm day or as a delightful dessert after a light dinner. This refreshing and creamy pie captures the classic root beer float flavor in a diabetic-friendly version.

Tropical Mango Popsicles

- **Preparation Time:** 10 minutes
- **Serves**: 6

Ingredients:

- 2 large ripe mangoes, peeled and diced

- 1 cup Greek yogurt (unsweetened)
- 1 tablespoon honey
- 1/2 cup coconut milk
- 1 teaspoon lime zest
- 2 tablespoons lime juice

Nutritional Information: Calories: 80 | Protein: 3g | Carbohydrates: 15g | Fat: 1.5g | Fiber: 2g

Instructions:

1. In a blender, puree diced mangoes until smooth.
2. In a bowl, combine Greek yogurt, honey (or sugar substitute), coconut milk, lime zest, and lime juice. Mix until well combined.
3. Layer the mango puree and yogurt mixture into popsicle molds.
4. Insert popsicle sticks and freeze for at least 4 hours or until fully set.
5. Run the molds under warm water for a few seconds to release the popsicles before serving.

Serving Suggestions:

- Enjoy Tropical Mango Popsicles as a guilt-free dessert or a refreshing snack on a hot day. These fruity popsicles offer a taste of the tropics with the sweetness of mango and a hint of lime, making them a delightful treat for all occasions.

Peppermint Meringues

- **Preparation Time:** 15 minutes
- **Serves:** 20 meringues

Ingredients:

1. 3 large egg whites
2. 3/4 cup powdered erythritol (or another sugar substitute)
3. 1/2 teaspoon peppermint extract
4. A pinch of cream of tartar
5. Sugar-free chocolate chips for garnish (optional)

Nutritional Information: Calories: 10 | Protein: 0g | Carbohydrates: 2g | Fat: 0g | Fiber: 0g

Instructions:

1. Preheat the oven to 200°F (95°C). Line a baking sheet with parchment paper.

2. In a clean, dry bowl, beat egg whites with a pinch of cream of tartar until soft peaks form.
3. Gradually add powdered erythritol, continuing to beat until stiff peaks form.
4. Gently fold in peppermint extract, being careful not to deflate the meringue.
5. Transfer the meringue mixture to a piping bag and pipe small swirls onto the prepared baking sheet.
6. Optionally, place a few sugar-free chocolate chips on top of each meringue.
7. Bake for 1.5 to 2 hours or until the meringues are crisp and dry.
8. Allow the meringues to cool completely before serving.

Serving Suggestions:

- Serve Peppermint Meringues as a light and airy dessert or a festive snack during the holiday season. These sugar-free treats provide a burst of peppermint flavor without compromising on the delicate and crisp texture of traditional meringues.

Low-Carb Trail Mix

- **Preparation Time:** 10 minutes
- **Serves:** 8

Ingredients:

- 1 cup almonds, unsalted
- 1/2 cup walnuts, unsalted
- 1/4 cup pumpkin seeds (pepitas)
- 1/4 cup sunflower seeds
- 1/4 cup unsweetened coconut flakes
- 1/4 cup dark chocolate chips (sugar-free)
- 1/4 cup dried cranberries (unsweetened)
- 1/2 teaspoon cinnamon
- 1/4 teaspoon sea salt

Nutritional Information: Calories: 180 | Protein: 6g | Carbohydrates: 8g | Fat: 15g | Fiber: 4g

Instructions:

1. In a large bowl, combine almonds, walnuts, pumpkin seeds, sunflower seeds, coconut flakes, dark chocolate chips, and dried cranberries.
2. Sprinkle cinnamon and sea salt over the mixture.
3. Toss the ingredients together until well combined.
4. Divide the trail mix into individual serving portions.

Serving Suggestions:

Enjoy Low-Carb Trail Mix as a convenient and satisfying snack between meals or on-the-go.

Ginger Plum Tart

- **Preparation Time:** 20 minutes
- **Serves**: 8

Ingredients:

- 1 pre-made low-carb pie crust
- 4 ripe plums, sliced
- 1/4 cup sugar substitute (erythritol or another suitable option)
- 1 teaspoon ground ginger
- 1 tablespoon almond flour
- 1/4 cup sliced almonds

- Sugar-free whipped cream for serving (optional)

Nutritional Information: Calories: 150 | Protein: 2g | Carbohydrates: 15g | Fat: 10g | Fiber: 4g

Instructions:

1. Preheat the oven according to the pie crust instructions.
2. Roll out the pie crust and press it into a tart pan.
3. In a bowl, toss sliced plums with sugar substitute, ground ginger, and almond flour.
4. Arrange the plum slices in the prepared tart crust.
5. Sprinkle sliced almonds over the plums.
6. Bake according to the pie crust instructions or until the plums are tender.
7. Allow the tart to cool before slicing.
8. Serve with a dollop of sugar-free whipped cream if desired.

Serving Suggestions:

- Indulge in the flavorful and aromatic Ginger Plum Tart as a sophisticated dessert after dinner.

Beverages/Drinks for Diabetic Gastroparesis Diet

Cinny Tea

- **Preparation Time**: 10 minutes
- **Serves**: 2

Ingredients:

- 2 cinnamon sticks
- 2 cups hot water
- 1 teaspoon black tea leaves
- 1 tablespoon sugar substitute (erythritol or another suitable option)

Nutritional Information: Calories: 0 | Protein: 0g | Carbohydrates: 0g | Fat: 0g | Fiber: 0g

Instructions:

1. In a teapot, place the cinnamon sticks.
2. Pour hot water over the cinnamon sticks and let them steep for 5 minutes.

3. Add black tea leaves to the pot and steep for an additional 3-4 minutes.
4. Strain the tea into cups, discarding the cinnamon sticks and tea leaves.
5. Optionally, sweeten with a sugar substitute if desired.
6. Serve hot and enjoy the comforting warmth of Cinny Tea.

Serving Suggestions:

- Cinny Tea is a delightful, caffeine-free beverage perfect for cozy evenings. Pair it with a splash of almond milk for added creaminess or enjoy it as is for a soothing, aromatic experience.

Pumpkin Latte

- **Preparation Time:** 15 minutes
- **Serves**: 2

Ingredients:

- 1 cup unsweetened almond milk
- 1/4 cup canned pumpkin puree

- 1 tablespoon sugar substitute (erythritol or another suitable option)
- 1/2 teaspoon pumpkin spice blend
- 1/2 cup strong brewed coffee or espresso
- Sugar-free whipped cream for topping (optional)

Nutritional Information: Calories: 30 | Protein: 1g | Carbohydrates: 3g | Fat: 2g | Fiber: 1g

Instructions:

1. In a small saucepan, heat almond milk, pumpkin puree, sugar substitute, and pumpkin spice blend over medium heat.
2. Whisk the mixture until it's well combined and heated through but not boiling.
3. Brew strong coffee or espresso separately.
4. Divide the coffee between two mugs.
5. Pour the pumpkin mixture over the coffee.
6. Optionally, top with sugar-free whipped cream.
7. Stir gently and enjoy the comforting flavors of Pumpkin Latte.

Serving Suggestions:

- Pumpkin Latte is a perfect autumn treat. Pair it with a sprinkle of cinnamon or nutmeg for an extra burst of flavor. This low-calorie, diabetes-friendly latte is a delicious alternative to traditional coffee shop offerings.

Mojito Mocktails

- **Preparation Time:** 10 minutes
- **Serves:** 2

Ingredients:

- 1 cup fresh mint leaves
- 1 tablespoon sugar substitute (erythritol or another suitable option)
- 1 lime, juiced
- 1/2 cup unsweetened lime-flavored sparkling water
- Ice cubes
- Fresh mint sprigs for garnish

Nutritional Information: Calories: 5 | Protein: 0g | Carbohydrates: 2g | Fat: 0g | Fiber: 1g

Instructions:

1. In a glass, muddle fresh mint leaves with sugar substitute.
2. Add lime juice to the glass and stir to combine.
3. Fill the glass with ice cubes.
4. Pour unsweetened lime-flavored sparkling water over the ice.
5. Stir gently to mix the flavors.
6. Garnish with fresh mint sprigs.
7. Serve immediately and savor the refreshing taste of Mojito Mocktails.

Serving Suggestions:

- Mojito Mocktails are a delightful non-alcoholic option, enjoy them on a sunny afternoon or as a crisp and satisfying beverage during warm evenings.

Dandy Chai

- **Preparation Time:** 15 minutes
- **Serves:** 2

Ingredients:

- 2 cups unsweetened almond milk
- 2 tablespoons roasted dandelion root tea
- 1 teaspoon ground cinnamon

- 1/2 teaspoon ground ginger
- 1/4 teaspoon ground cardamom
- 1 tablespoon sugar substitute (erythritol or another suitable option)
- A pinch of black pepper (optional)

Nutritional Information: Calories: 15 | Protein: 1g | Carbohydrates: 2g | Fat: 1g | Fiber: 1g

Instructions:

1. In a small saucepan, heat almond milk until it's warm but not boiling.
2. Add roasted dandelion root tea, ground cinnamon, ground ginger, ground cardamom, and sugar substitute to the saucepan.
3. Simmer the mixture over low heat for 10 minutes, allowing the flavors to meld.
4. Strain the tea into cups, removing tea leaves.
5. Add a pinch of black pepper if desired.
6. Stir well and enjoy the unique taste of Dandy Chai.

Serving Suggestions:

- Dandy Chai is a caffeine-free alternative with earthy notes. Pair it with a cinnamon stick or a sprinkle of cinnamon on top for added warmth and flavor. This herbal chai is a cozy and comforting beverage for any time of the day.

Rooibos Tea

- **Preparation Time:** 5 minutes
- **Serves:** 2

Ingredients:

- 2 rooibos tea bags
- 2 cups hot water
- 1 tablespoon sugar substitute (erythritol or another suitable option)
- Fresh lemon slices for garnish

Nutritional Information: Calories: 0 | Protein: 0g | Carbohydrates: 0g | Fat: 0g | Fiber: 0g

Instructions:

1. Place rooibos tea bags in a teapot.
2. Pour hot water over the tea bags and let them steep for 3-5 minutes, remove the tea bags and discard them.

3. Stir in sugar substitute until dissolved.
4. Pour the tea into cups.
5. Garnish with fresh lemon slices.
6. Enjoy the mild and soothing flavor of Rooibos Tea.

Serving Suggestions:

- Rooibos Tea, also known as red bush tea, is caffeine-free and rich in antioxidants. Pair it with a slice of lemon for a citrusy twist or enjoy it plain for a calming and hydrating experience.

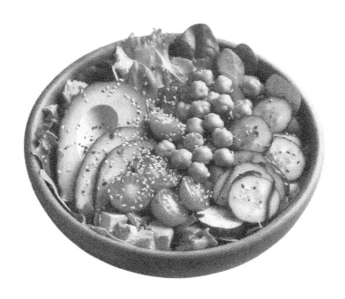

CHAPTER 3

30 Days Meal Plan For Diabetic Gastroparesis Diet

Please note that the provided meal plan is a sample and should not be interpreted as a recommendation to consume all the listed recipes in a single day.

This meal plan aims to offer inspiration and guidance for healthy meal preparation. Feel free to customize this plan to suit your preferences and dietary requirements.

Day 1

- **Breakfast:** White Cheddar Zucchini Muffins
- **Lunch:** Tuna Teriyaki Kabobs
- **Dinner:** Feta Garbanzo Bean Salad
- **Snack:** Root Beer Float Pie

Day 2:

- **Breakfast:** Pumpkin Latte
- **Lunch:** Garlic Tilapia with Spicy Kale
- **Dinner:** Skillet Sea Scallops

- **Snack:** Tropical Mango Popsicles

Day 3:

- **Breakfast:** Mojito Mocktails
- **Lunch:** Shrimp Orzo with Feta
- **Dinner:** Carne Asada Tacos
- **Snack:** Peppermint Meringues

Day 4:

- **Breakfast:** Dandy Chai
- **Lunch:** Fish Tacos with Guacamole
- **Dinner:** Green Goddess Salad with Chickpeas
- **Snack:** Low-Carb Trail Mix

Day 5:

- **Breakfast:** Rooibos Tea
- **Lunch:** Caprese Sandwich
- **Dinner:** Asian Lettuce Wraps
- **Snack:** Ginger Plum Tart

Day 6:

- **Breakfast:** Mini Corn, Cheese, and Basil Frittatas
- **Lunch:** Artichoke Ratatouille Chicken

- **Dinner:** Beef and Spinach Lo Mein
- **Snack:** Chocolate-Dipped Strawberries with Almonds

Day 7:

- **Breakfast:** Vegetarian Eggs and Lentils on Toast
- **Lunch:** Egg Salad Lettuce Wraps
- **Dinner:** Hamburger Vegetable Soup
- **Snack:** Chia Seed and Berry Parfait

Day 8:

- **Breakfast:** Cinny Tea
- **Lunch:** Tuna Teriyaki Kabobs
- **Dinner:** Feta Garbanzo Bean Salad
- **Snack:** Root Beer Float Pie

Day 9:

- **Breakfast:** Pumpkin Latte
- **Lunch:** Garlic Tilapia with Spicy Kale
- **Dinner:** Skillet Sea Scallops
- **Snack:** Tropical Mango Popsicles

Day 10:

- **Breakfast:** Mojito Mocktails
- **Lunch:** Shrimp Orzo with Feta
- **Dinner:** Carne Asada Tacos
- **Snack:** Peppermint Meringues

Day 11:

- **Breakfast:** Dandy Chai
- **Lunch:** Fish Tacos with Guacamole
- **Dinner:** Green Goddess Salad with Chickpeas
- **Snack:** Low-Carb Trail Mix

Day 12:

- **Breakfast:** Rooibos Tea
- **Lunch:** Caprese Sandwich
- **Dinner:** Asian Lettuce Wraps
- **Snack:** Ginger Plum Tart

Day 13:

- **Breakfast:** Mini Corn, Cheese, and Basil Frittatas
- **Lunch:** Artichoke Ratatouille Chicken
- **Dinner:** Beef and Spinach Lo Mein

- **Snack:** Chocolate-Dipped Strawberries with Almonds

Day 14:

- **Breakfast:** Vegetarian Eggs and Lentils on Toast
- **Lunch:** Egg Salad Lettuce Wraps
- **Dinner:** Hamburger Vegetable Soup
- **Snack:** Chia Seed and Berry Parfait

Day 15:

- **Breakfast:** Cinny Tea
- **Lunch:** Tuna Teriyaki Kabobs
- **Dinner:** Feta Garbanzo Bean Salad
- **Snack:** Root Beer Float Pie

Day 16:

- **Breakfast:** Pumpkin Latte
- **Lunch:** Garlic Tilapia with Spicy Kale
- **Dinner:** Skillet Sea Scallops
- **Snack:** Tropical Mango Popsicles

Day 17:

- **Breakfast:** Mojito Mocktails

- **Lunch:** Shrimp Orzo with Feta
- **Dinner:** Carne Asada Tacos
- **Snack:** Peppermint Meringues

Day 18:

- **Breakfast:** Dandy Chai
- **Lunch:** Fish Tacos with Guacamole
- **Dinner:** Green Goddess Salad with Chickpeas
- **Snack:** Low-Carb Trail Mix

Day 19:

- **Breakfast:** Rooibos Tea
- **Lunch:** Caprese Sandwich
- **Dinner:** Asian Lettuce Wraps
- **Snack:** Ginger Plum Tart

Day 20:

- **Breakfast:** Mini Corn, Cheese, and Basil Frittatas
- **Lunch:** Artichoke Ratatouille Chicken
- **Dinner:** Beef and Spinach Lo Mein
- **Snack:** Chocolate-Dipped Strawberries with Almonds

Day 21:

- **Breakfast:** Vegetarian Eggs and Lentils on Toast
- **Lunch:** Egg Salad Lettuce Wraps
- **Dinner:** Hamburger Vegetable Soup
- **Snack:** Chia Seed and Berry Parfait

Day 22:

- **Breakfast:** Cinny Tea
- **Lunch:** Tuna Teriyaki Kabobs
- **Dinner:** Feta Garbanzo Bean Salad
- **Snack:** Root Beer Float Pie

Day 23:

- **Breakfast:** Pumpkin Latte
- **Lunch:** Garlic Tilapia with Spicy Kale
- **Dinner:** Skillet Sea Scallops
- **Snack:** Tropical Mango Popsicles

Day 24:

- **Breakfast:** Mojito Mocktails
- **Lunch:** Shrimp Orzo with Feta
- **Dinner:** Carne Asada Tacos

- **Snack:** Peppermint Meringues

Day 25:

- **Breakfast:** Dandy Chai
- **Lunch:** Fish Tacos with Guacamole
- **Dinner:** Green Goddess Salad with Chickpeas
- **Snack:** Low-Carb Trail Mix

Day 26:

- **Breakfast:** Rooibos Tea
- **Lunch:** Caprese Sandwich
- **Dinner:** Asian Lettuce Wraps
- **Snack:** Ginger Plum Tart

Day 27:

- **Breakfast:** Mini Corn, Cheese, and Basil Frittatas
- **Lunch:** Artichoke Ratatouille Chicken
- **Dinner:** Beef and Spinach Lo Mein
- **Snack:** Chocolate-Dipped Strawberries with Almonds

Day 28:

- **Breakfast:** Vegetarian Eggs and Lentils on Toast

- **Lunch:** Egg Salad Lettuce Wraps
- **Dinner:** Hamburger Vegetable Soup
- **Snack:** Chia Seed and Berry Parfait

Day 29:

- **Breakfast:** Cinny Tea
- **Lunch:** Tuna Teriyaki Kabobs
- **Dinner:** Feta Garbanzo Bean Salad
- **Snack:** Root Beer Float Pie

Day 30:

- **Breakfast:** Pumpkin Latte
- **Lunch:** Garlic Tilapia with Spicy Kale
- **Dinner:** Skillet Sea Scallops
- **Snack:** Tropical Mango Popsicles

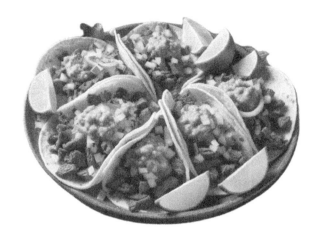

CHAPTER 4

Conclusion

In closing, "The Diabetic Gastroparesis Diet Cookbook" offers not just a collection of recipes but a holistic guide to navigating the challenges of managing diabetic gastroparesis through mindful and flavorful eating.

This journey through nourishment is not merely about restriction but about embracing a renewed relationship with food, one that prioritizes health without compromising on taste.

As we conclude this culinary expedition, it's crucial to recognize the empowering principles that underpin this cookbook.

The benefits of this diet extend beyond mere sustenance. By understanding and implementing the carefully curated principles within these pages, you are not only addressing the specific challenges of gastroparesis but also fostering overall well-being.

The incorporation of wholesome ingredients, thoughtful meal planning, and the avoidance of problematic foods contribute to a lifestyle that supports not just physical health but also a positive relationship with food.

The comprehensive meal plan, spanning breakfast to dessert and beverages, provides a roadmap for a month-long culinary exploration. The diverse array of recipes ensures that each day is met with excitement, as you savor the rich tapestry of flavors while adhering to the guidelines of the Diabetic Gastroparesis Diet.

In the spirit of culinary adventure, this cookbook invites you to experiment with new ingredients, textures, and combinations. It encourages a shift from viewing dietary restrictions as limitations to embracing them as opportunities for creativity and discovery in the kitchen.

As you embark on your personal journey with this cookbook, remember that each meal is a chance to nourish not only the body but also the spirit.

With these recipes, may you find joy in the kitchen, savor every bite, and discover that managing diabetic gastroparesis can be a flavorful and fulfilling experience.

Here's to vibrant health and the endless possibilities that a well-crafted, mindful diet can bring to your table.

Made in the USA
Monee, IL
27 June 2024

60819968R00049